Bubble tea chain

The best teas for discontinuous fasting

DREW FORD

Table contents

What Is Discontinuous Fasting

Discontinuous fasting is a dietary method and direction for living. It includes cycling eating and fasting windows during explicit time periods. There are a few different fasting strategies, including 5:2, 16:8, and eat-stop-eat. The 5:2 technique empowers you to eat normally for five days out of the week. The excess two days are fasting days, where you eat simply 500 to 600 calories all day long.

The 16/8 strategy includes eating the whole day's calories in 8 hours and fasting for the other 16 hours. A large portion of these techniques advocate eating between early afternoon and 8 p.m. and afterward setting the fasting window from 8 p.m. to early afternoon the next day.

The eat-stop-eat strategy includes limiting all food utilization for 24-hour durations several times each week. These irregular fasting techniques are intended to start up digestion, increment energy, and advance, generally speaking, better wellbeing. The following are a couple of the medical advantages of irregular fasting.

The most effective method to make Quick With Tea

The expression "discontinuous fasting" has become very famous as of late with benefits like weight reduction, stable glucose levels, decreased hazard of cardiovascular illness, and upgrades with other medical issues. Luckily, tea can be utilized to make your irregular fasting more charming and, surprisingly, more powerful. The Craft of Tea has an assortment of free-leaf teas, tea assortments, and flavors to help your energy and temperament while fasting.

What's so perfect about fasting

Discontinuous fasting has positive medical advantages, and it's very easy to stick with, making it reasonable over the long haul. Whether you are hoping to shed a couple of pounds, work on your overall wellbeing, or lift your energy levels, discontinuous fasting with tea can help. There are straightforward principles with irregular fasting: you want to separate your time into an eating time and a non-eating time. Contingent upon your objectives and way of life, there are maybe a couple approaches to an irregular fasting diet. You could decide to fast in light of the days, for instance, eating one day and not eating the following. Or, on the other hand, you could decide to be quick in view of the hours in a day. Commonly, the most utilized plan is eating for 8 hours and fasting for 16 hours (the vast majority of which you are snoozing for).

Advantages of Discontinuous Fasting with Tea

Tea improves discontinuous fasting and is, by and large, simpler. Despite the fact that you might be limiting the time you can eat, you can constantly have some relieving tea while rehearsing the eating routine. At Specialty of Tea, we accept that the advantages of fasting with tea are interminable, but these are the main benefits:

Feed Your Yearning: During the fasting time span, it might take your stomach a couple of days to become accustomed to feeling lighter and not processing food constantly. You will likewise begin to feel very ravenous during these periods. We suggest you feed your body with tea. Green tea is known to calm food cravings and reduce any inconvenience while fasting.Feel Quiet: For a quieting soul, the best teas to brew with are ginger and hibiscus. These teas will uphold your energy levels, however, they won't leave you feeling jumpy like the caffeine in some espresso. All things being equal, you can remain composed, careful, and centered all through your fast.Support Your Body's Wellbeing: Tea leaves contain polyphenols, which are strong cell reinforcements that can assist with stomach-related wellbeing, more splendid and more clear skin, and an upgraded center. While all tea leaves can give you these advantages, while practicing irregular fasting, we suggest green tea, ginger, and hibiscus for the best outcomes.

BEST TEAS TO Quickly With

Discontinuous fasting with tea is tied into figuring out how your body feels and how to address any distress you are feeling. Eventually, you ought to pick teas that you enjoy, are really great for your body, and will assist you in getting past the fasting stage. For a little assistance, the Craft of Tea suggests fasting with ginger, hibiscus, and green tea. Ginger tea can assist with calming a resentful or touchy stomach. It likewise has an extraordinary, solid flavor that guides in quieting your state of mind and feelings. Attempt our Excited Turmeric Ginger Tea for this definite reason. Hibiscus tea is perfect for its calming impact. We suggest drinking some hibiscus tea by the day's end, prior to hitting the sack, to reset your brain and have a decent night's rest. Green tea has for quite some time been utilized to help with weight reduction while additionally supporting energy. It can assist you with traversing the harder times of fasting by encouraging you in any event when you haven't eaten.
Attempt irregular fasting with tea today!
Assuming you are keen on discontinuous fasting, why not start today? We urge you to glance through our tea items and find flavors and blends that you love, which will help you through this excursion. Assuming you have any inquiries or need help, kindly make sure to join the Craft of Tea group. We wish you sure energy as you start your discontinuous fasting with tea.

The best teas for discontinuous fasting

During fasting, ensure your tea contains no added substances that will break your fast. These incorporate organic products, sugars (for example, stevia), or flavors. Here are our top choices:

Green tea contains catechins and caffeine, which both make an antioxidative difference (i.e., are cell-defensive) and invigorate your digestion.Dark tea comes from a similar plant (Camellia sinensis). It contrasts, be that as it may, in the handling of the leaves and its typical caffeine content.Natural tea can have various properties depending on the variety, yet by and large it has a quieting, stomach-related invigorating, and vitalizing impact.Ginger tea upholds your absorption and susceptibility framework.

Three ways to appreciate tea in a sound manner

Consume caffeine with some restraint! A lot of caffeine can hold you back from dozing and can set glycogen free from the liver, causing your insulin levels to rise.Favor natural, free tea leaves! These have more supplements and a superior taste.Partake in your tea, cold-brewed. This protects more important fixings. Also, particularly in summer, this is exceptionally revitalizing!This is the manner in which you can help your irregular fasting with tea. A decent cup of tea is not exclusively tasty, but it also upholds the constructive outcomes of irregular fasting. In this manner, you get in shape effectively and support your wellbeing and prosperity.

How Tea Can Improve Your Outcomes

Irregular fasting is a famous pattern for wellbeing. It draws on transformative practices and offers tools that incorporate expanded energy and further develop wellbeing. It's regularly coordinated with other dietary changes, including the ketogenic diet (keto).
You don't need to burn through a lot of cash on extravagant, irregular fasts. Truth be told, you can essentially mix up your #1 cup of tea and integrate it into your fasting plan. Peruse on to figure out how and find some incredible fasting tea thoughts to attempt today. Need to get some irregular fasting tea today? Look at our assortment of the best teas to supplement your irregular fasting plan here.

Advantages of Irregular Fasting Tea

Sped up weight reduction

The main cooperation with irregular fasting for some individuals happens as they search for ways of getting in shape quicker. Research shows that discontinuous fasting might assist with expanding fat copying by diminishing insulin levels

That is on the grounds that insulin influences the manner in which the body retains glucose, which it then, at that point, changes over into fat stores or consumes as energy.

A meta-examination distributed in subatomic and cell endocrinology looks at d40 and zeros in on weight reduction and energy limitations. Scientists observed that irregular fasting was a substantial choice for individuals who were hoping to diminish muscle mass versus fat and get in shape

A subsequent report distributed by JAMA Interior Medication examined the effects of substitute day fasting on weight reduction and weight maintenance. The randomized clinical preliminary consisted of 100 metabolically solid, hefty people who were observed for a one-year time frame. Specialists found that other day fasting and day-to-day calorie limitation were similarly compelling, contrasted with a fake treatment in overseeing weight and speeding up weight reduction

Irregular fasting might be easier to oversee for individuals who are hoping to get in shape when contrasted with calorie limitation. That is on the grounds that you can in any case eat anything you desire; you simply need to do it within a specific time span. Calorie limitations require denying yourself specific food sources or restricting your intake, which can feel less satisfying and more troublesome while attempting to shed pounds.

further developed heart wellbeing

Irregular fasting might assist with supporting heart wellbeing by bringing down circulatory strain, fatty oils, and awful LDL cholesterol. A survey distributed in 2017 found that gorging might prompt insulin obstruction, overabundance fat, and cardiovascular illness, particularly when combined with a stationary way of life. The investigation discovered that discontinuous fasting could assist with decreasing these dangers and further develop weight reduction

Better Cerebrum Capability

Irregular fasting doesn't simply support energy; it can likewise assist with working on your concentration and readiness. A creature study published in PLOS analyzed the impact of discontinuous fasting on the mental capabilities of mice. Scientists observed that mice that benefited from an irregular fasting premise exhibited better learning capacities and memory abilities

decreased chance of diabetes

The medical advantages of irregular fasting extend likewise to infection counteraction. Type 2 diabetes is a condition where the body can't create sufficient insulin or experiences issues handling it—otherwise called insulin responsiveness. A review distributed in Translational Exploration analyzed the impacts of irregular fasting and substitute day fasting on type 2 diabetes risk. Specialists found that fasting assisted the body with consuming fat quicker and brought about critical weight reduction compared with fake treatment. Scientists likewise found that fasting brought about lower levels of insulin resistance, lower glucose levels, and fasting insulin

How Tea Further Develops Irregular Fasting Results

Ends Craving

Many individuals battle with cravings for food during the initial few days or long stretches of discontinuous fasting. That is on the grounds that your body is accustomed to having nourishment for energy over the course of the day. Drinking tea can assist with facilitating these issues as your body adjusts to the fasting time frame.

A review published in Clinical Sustenance found that catechins in tea hinder the emission of ghrelin, the chemical responsible for flagging the sensation of craving. These green tea catechins incorporate EGCG, or epigallocatechin gallate, a cell reinforcement responsible for a large number of tea's medical advantages, including the rummaging of free revolutionaries Drinking tea can assist you with slipping into the fasting experience while treating a portion of the normal incidental effects or changing your dietary patterns. On a substance level, drinking tea can assist with obstructing the craving chemical by diminishing ghrelin levels, stopping hunger in its tracks.

Helps with weight reduction results

There is broad examination showing that drinking tea might assist with speeding up weight reduction while additionally assisting with overseeing weight over the long haul. Tea is a calorie-free drink, making it an incredible substitution for juices and diet soft drinks on the off chance that you're checking your calorie intake.

Beside that, catechins in tea help to increase fat misfortune. One way tea does this is by raising the body's inside temperature. Caffeine likewise attempts to increase energy consumption and fat oxidation, helping you shed pounds quicker

Helps Detox

Drinking tea alongside irregular fasting assists the body's regular detox through a process known as autophagy. The cycle is set off by the initiation of a protein, which urges the body to flush out damaged cells and empowers the recovery of new cells. This cycle is fundamental with regards to protecting bulk and forestalling age-related infections.

During the fasting window, tea catechins activate autophagy, helping the body detox and revamp cells

The catechins in tea additionally help to dispense with free radicals that can cause oxidative pressure. Oxidative pressure is the body's type of rust and has for quite some time been connected to degenerative illnesses that incorporate untimely maturing.

Supports Unwinding

Drinking tea is additionally perfect for cerebral wellbeing, very much like discontinuous fasting. The mitigating demonstration of drinking tea can assist you with loosening up following an unpleasant day and permit you to take a couple of moments to zero in on your own wellbeing. Drinking tea has likewise been shown to assist with diminishing feelings of anxiety by hindering the stress chemical cortisol

The Best Irregular Fasting Teas to Attempt

1. Green Tea

Green tea is a solid mixture that is a staple of the weight reduction industry. It's sold in a concentrated form as green tea pills that assist in weight reduction. The tea is likewise an incredible method for expanding your fasting benefits.

Concentrates show that green tea increments the metabolic rate and can help 24-hour energy use by very nearly 5% (11). That implies you can consume fat quicker and arrive at your weight reduction objectives sooner. The catechins in green tea additionally help to bring down levels of appetite chemicals to keep you feeling full after your last feast—in any event, during longer diets.

2. Ginger tea

Ginger tea is a fantastic natural tea to add to your fasting regimen. It's eminent for its stomach-related medical advantages, which include decreasing sickness side effects and supporting the body for the breakdown of food (12). A review published in Digestion found ginger improves thermogenesis, a characteristic body process that helps ignite fat burning. Scientists likewise viewed that as ginger assisting with diminishing sensations of appetite. That implies you can remain focused on your fasting plan and eat only during the eating window.

3. Rooibos Tea

Rooibos tea is another homegrown tea that is normally sans caffeine, making it an extraordinary tea to savor the nights. Rooibos tea is prestigious for its liver-health benefits. As far as fasting support, rooibos tea can assist the body with processing fat all the more proficiently.

A review published in Phytomedicine examined the impacts of rooibos tea on weight. In the in vitro study, specialists found that rooibos tea prevented the arrangement of fat cells and helped digestion.

4. Dark Tea

Dark tea is produced using a similar plant as green teas. The leaves are permitted to oxidize for an extensive stretch of time, which turns the leaves a profoundly dark shade and imparts a strong flavor like dark espresso. It contains about a portion of how much caffeine is in a standard mug of espresso, yet it likewise contains an amino acid known as L-theanine. This amino acid eases back the arrival of caffeine, bringing about a more extended and enduring jolt of energy and an expanded center. This supplements the advantages of fasting.

Support fasting results with tea

For the best outcomes, specialists prescribe drinking 3 to 4 cups of tea every day to support the advantages of fasting. For the most extreme effect, attempt cold blending your tea. Cold-fermented tea contains a larger number of cell reinforcements than customarily soaked tea. That is on the grounds that the high-temperature water can consume a portion of the catechins and cell reinforcements.

The virus blend process includes soaking the tea leaves in cool water for a longer period of time. Ordinarily, the leaves ought to soak in the cool water for eight to twelve hours. Hold back nothing of the free leaves for each eight ounces of water.

In the event that you're hoping to oversee body weight or increment weight reduction, irregular fasting is an extraordinary method for accomplishing your objectives. Drinking tea can assist with expanding the advantages of fasting. It likewise offers a large group of medical advantages that lift the invulnerable framework and advance general prosperity.

A Manual for Tea and Fasting

Green tea is one of many, many types of teas accessible at this moment, and many are showcased for their helpful and medical advantages.

Notwithstanding, for this article, we'll separate these teas into two classes: customary teas (green tea analogs) and different teas.

There are four sorts of conventional teas, each taken from the leaves of the Camellia sinensis plant:

White tea

Green tea (or matcha)

Oolong tea

Dark tea

The primary contrast between every one of these teas is the way the leaves are aged, which changes the densities of their cell reinforcements, flavonoids, and caffeine. Subsequently, these types of tea can be considered to have comparable advantages to green tea from a wide perspective, yet their singular impacts can have changing qualities.

Different teas, similar to natural teas and organic product teas, come from different plants and spices. Instances of different teas include:

Homegrown tea

Peppermint tea

Hibiscus tea

Chamomile tea

Rooibos tea

Ginger tea

While a significant number of these teas have fantastic medical advantages thanks to catechins and other cell reinforcement compounds, they're not close to as beneficial as the four traditional teas from Camellia sinensis.

Refreshments to Drink While Irregularly Fasting

Most conventional and homegrown teas are fantastic beverages while discontinuous fasting, and we've likewise incorporated a few different choices that can keep you full and invigorated, check your craving, taste perfect, and may try and speed up weight reduction.

So which are the best beverages while discontinuous fasting?

Water

Carbonated water

Natural teas

Green tea

Green juices (produced using verdant green and non-boring vegetables)

Apple juice and vinegar

The Last Word on Green Tea Fasting

As we've addressed above, intermittent fasting has a large number of advantages, both for weight loss and general wellbeing.

Also, green tea has comparative impacts, which makes it the ideal beverage to control your craving during your fasting windows.

We additionally talked about how other customary teas can make comparable impacts. Homegrown teas and natural product teas are additionally great choices; however, their characteristics can change beyond what we investigate in this article.

Amla Green takes each of the advantages of green tea and adds the advantages of amla (which is seemingly the most impressive restorative plant on earth) without breaking your quick.

To dive deeper into one of the most intense normal beverages for discontinuous fasting and attempt your most memorable cluster sans risk, click beneath.

To study one of the most intense normal beverages for discontinuous fasting and attempt your most memorable group sans risk, click beneath.

Amla Green is accessible in both ordinary and decaffeinated forms, and it furthermore arrives in a delectably reviving hibiscus flavor. Attempt one today!

What is panda

Pandan is a sweet-smelling plant that is generally utilized in South and Southeast Asian food. It has a sweet botanical scent for food. Furthermore, pandan leaves mixed with tea make a fascinating beverage. Pandan tea is the most beloved drink of numerous Vietnamese individuals. All in all, what makes this sort of tea extraordinary?

What is pandan tea

Tea blended from dried pandan leaves has a sweet taste and fragrance. It is an imaginative kind of tea because of its extraordinary flavor and nutritious characteristics. The fundamental element of pandan tea is the utilization of an enormous amount of tea buds in the mix, which is a mark of a great tea. Pandan tea tastes very herbal and new, yet in addition it has a great deal of medical advantages.

What sort of Vietnamese pandan tea does FGC give

Mixed panda tea (with dried natural products or with herbals)

This pandan tea is made by mixing tea leaves with pandan leaves, as per one of a kind seasoning techniques. Due to utilizing an enormous number of tea buds, pandan tea is a top-notch tea with a herby and new taste. The tea will get some margin to blend, however, and has a more extravagant desire and smell, making for an incredible encounter for shoppers.

pandan tea powder

As per clients' requirements, FGC can create pandan tea powder with the principal fixings, for example, pandan leaves, green tea, and so on. These fixings are blended in a specific proportion and ground into a fine powder. While making tea, you simply have to soak the powder in scalding hot water and appreciate it.

Moment Pandan Tea

Moment Pandan tea is created using the advanced handling strategy for FGC. The tea is an ideal mix of pandan extricate, tea remove, and different fixings, for example, jasmine separate, and so on. Moment tea effectively disintegrates in water, is easy to make, yet at the same time holds its flavor. It tends to be a reasonable beverage for the comfort of buyers.

RTD Pandan Tea

The fundamental elements of RTD Pandan tea from FGC are green tea, pandan leaves cut, jasmine bloom, and spices. Our RTD tea is a protected and sound drink, with numerous food-safe acknowledgments and certificates. The method for safeguarding it is simple and does not influence the quality. Accordingly, this sort of tea can be appreciated everywhere and whenever.

Pandan Tea

Pandan tea mixed with different spices is exceptionally famous for its medical advantages and rich flavors. This tea isn't just powerful in rewards, but additionally assists with advancing wellbeing and warding off a few sicknesses. Here is a portion of its medical advantages: forestall coronary illness

Pandan leaves contain carotenoids, a class of cellular reinforcements. These substances are known to lessen the risk of creating atherosclerosis, the limiting of the heart's conduits because of plaque development. In this way, pandan tea is known as a decent beverage for heart wellbeing.

Forestall disease

Pandan is an incredible wellspring of nutrients and cell reinforcements, which can assist with diminishing harmful free radicals. Besides, drinking pandan tea is likewise viewed as a method for supporting the safe framework and preventing malignant growth, coronary illness, and so on. That is the reason many individuals utilize this tea.

Control glucose

A few investigations have shown that pandan tea might control the glucose of consumers. Subsequent to drinking pandan tea, individuals had lower glucose than the ones who didn't drink it. Pandan's passing on may diminish and balance out glucose.

filter and detoxify the body.

Pandan tea likewise contains unadulterated micronutrients to help the body clear intensity and detoxify. Moreover, nutrients in pandan tea, like L-ascorbic acid, thiamin, and so forth, can reinforce opposition, cool, and delay skin maturation.

Fascinating realities about pandan

Pandan is a lasting spice that fills in heat and humidity. There are numerous subspecies of pandan. The spice is utilized in numerous ways, both in food and in assembly. Its buds are used as a fixing in cooking, while pandan leaves are a great flavor enhancer; obviously, it is also utilized for tea production.
In the same way as other things in Asia, pandan plants have an extraordinary conventional importance for the local people. The long, spiky branch goes out from negative energy and makes a place of refuge liberated from excluded visitors.
Tea produced using dried pandan leaves is an extraordinary tonic. It is an exceptionally invigorating tea with a herby smell, which people who love the delicate and light taste of this tea request.

Instructions to blend some panda tea

Above all else, the tea set ought to be pre-warmed with boiling water. Then, at that point, the tea leaves ought to be added to the tea kettle; the amount depends on taste.
The tea leaves ought to soak at 80 °C for 30 seconds before each cup is filled.
At last, the tea ought to be appreciated and delighted in. Pandan green tea can hold its flavor for quite a while. The tea might go cold, but the flavor will remain.
Note: To make unadulterated and wonderful tea, you ought to pour the water gradually and leave the top of the tea kettle open while not blending tea.

Conclusion

Pandan is a flexible plant with different culinary and restorative applications across South and Southeast Asia. It might assist with bringing down your glucose and assuage joint inflammation torment; however, more examination is required.
Its foods are grown from the ground; the sharp leaves are widely eaten and utilized in various dishes, lending an unmistakable variety and vanilla-like botanical notes.
On the off chance that it isn't regularly developed or sold in your area, search for powdered, separated, or frozen pandan leaves.

9 798374 564426